Adrenal Fatigue Syndrome Treatment Guide

Lifestyle Changes for Managing Adrenal Fatigue

By

Oren Kenny

Table of Contents

CHAPTER 1 7

Introduction to Adrenal Fatigue
Syndrome 7

   1.1 What is Adrenal Fatigue? 7

   1.2 Causes and Risk Factors of
Adrenal Fatigue Syndrome 13

   1.3 Recognizing the Symptoms of
Adrenal Fatigue Syndrome 18

CHAPTER 2 22

Understanding the Adrenal Glands and
their Functions...................................22

   2.1 Anatomy of the Adrenal Glands
....22

   2.2 The Role of Adrenal Hormones 24

   2.3 How Stress Affects Adrenal
Function 27

CHAPTER 3 30

Diagnosing Adrenal Fatigue Syndrome
....30

3.1 Medical History and Physical Examination 30

3.2 Saliva and Blood Tests for Adrenal Hormones: 32

3.3 Differentiating Adrenal Fatigue from Other Conditions 34

CHAPTER 4 37

Lifestyle Changes for Managing Adrenal Fatigue 37

4.1 Stress Management Techniques
....37

4.2 Sleep Optimization 39

4.3 Balanced Nutrition and Dietary Recommendations 41

4.4 Importance of Regular Exercise43

CHAPTER 5 45

Herbal and Nutritional Supplements for Adrenal Support.........................45

5.1 Adaptogenic Herbs 45

5.2 Vitamins and Minerals for Adrenal Health 48

5.3 Recommended Dosages and Precautions 50

CHAPTER 6 53

Prescription Medications for Adrenal Fatigue 53

6.1 Corticosteroids and their Use ... 53

6.2 Risks and Benefits of Medication 55

6.3 Monitoring and Adjusting Treatment 57

CHAPTER 7 60

Complementary Therapies for Adrenal Fatigue 60

7.1 Acupuncture and Acupressure .60

7.1.1 Acupuncture 61

7.1.2 Acupressure 61

7.2 Massage Therapy 62

7.3 Yoga and Meditation 65

7.3.1 Yoga....................................66

7.3.2 Meditation 66

7.4 Biofeedback and Relaxation Techniques 68

7.4.1 Relaxation Techniques 68

7.4.2 Biofeedback........................69

CHAPTER 8 71

Lifestyle Tips for Long-Term Adrenal Health 71

8.1 Creating a Supportive Environment....................................71

8.2 Building Resilience to Stress.....73

8.3 Monitoring Progress and Identifying Triggers........................74

CHAPTER 9 78

Adrenal Fatigue in Special Populations 78

9.1 Adrenal Fatigue in Women.......78

9.2 Adrenal Fatigue in Men 82

CHAPTER 10 86

Seeking Professional Help and Finding the Right Specialist 86

10.1 Choosing the Right Healthcare Provider 86

10.2 Questions to Ask During Consultations 91

CHAPTER 11 96

How Long Does Recovery from Adrenal Fatigue Take?...................................96

CHAPTER 12 101

Empowering Yourself for Recovery .101

CHAPTER 1

Introduction to Adrenal Fatigue Syndrome

1.1 What is Adrenal Fatigue?

Adrenal Fatigue Syndrome is a term used to describe a collection of symptoms believed to be caused by an underactive adrenal gland or dysfunction of the hypothalamic-pituitary-adrenal (HPA) axis. This condition is controversial and not widely recognized by the conventional medical community, which has led to varying opinions on its validity and treatment. However, it has gained popularity in alternative and integrative medicine circles.

The adrenal glands, which are located above the kidneys, play a crucial role in the body's stress response and the regulation of several important hormones. One of their primary functions is to release hormones such as cortisol and adrenaline in response to stress, helping the body adapt and cope with various challenges.

The concept of Adrenal Fatigue suggests that chronic or prolonged stress can overwhelm the adrenal glands, leading to an inability to produce adequate levels of hormones. This purportedly results in a cascade of symptoms that affect various body systems, causing fatigue, among other issues.

It's important to note that the term "Adrenal Fatigue" is a bit not understandable because it implies that the adrenal glands are completely exhausted, similar to how a muscle might become fatigued after intense exercise. In reality, adrenal function is more complex, and the issue may involve dysregulation rather than complete exhaustion. This lack of precision in the term has contributed to skepticism among some medical professionals.

Symptoms commonly associated with Adrenal Fatigue Syndrome include:

1. Chronic Fatigue: A persistent feeling of tiredness, even after adequate rest and sleep. People with Adrenal Fatigue often report feeling exhausted and have difficulty getting through the day.

2. Sleep Disturbances: Insomnia or difficulty falling asleep or staying asleep is common in individuals with this condition. Disruptions in the body's natural circadian rhythm may lead to sleep issues.

3. Stress and Anxiety: Adrenal hormones play a role in the body's stress response, and imbalances can lead to increased feelings of stress and anxiety, as well as a reduced ability to cope with daily stressors.

4. Brain Fog and Memory Problems: Difficulty concentrating, poor memory, and cognitive challenges are frequently reported by those who believe they have Adrenal Fatigue.

5. Low Energy and Motivation: People with Adrenal Fatigue often

experience reduced energy levels and a lack of motivation to engage in regular activities.

6. Digestive Problems: Adrenal imbalances may contribute to digestive issues such as bloating, constipation, or diarrhea.

7. Changes in Weight: Some individuals may experience weight gain or difficulty losing weight due to hormonal imbalances affecting metabolism.

8. Low Blood Pressure: Adrenal hormones play a role in regulating blood pressure, and disruptions in this process can lead to low blood pressure in some cases.

9. Sensitivity to Cold: Individuals with Adrenal Fatigue might have difficulty staying warm and may feel cold more easily than others.

10. Reduced Immune Function: The stress-related impact on the immune system could lead to increased susceptibility to infections and a longer recovery time.

It is crucial to understand that these symptoms can be caused by various medical conditions and are not specific to Adrenal Fatigue. Many of the symptoms overlap with other health issues, making it challenging to diagnose Adrenal Fatigue definitively.

While some healthcare practitioners and individuals swear by the concept of Adrenal Fatigue and its treatment, others argue that the symptoms attributed to this condition are often nonspecific and could be explained by other underlying health problems.

It is essential to approach the topic of Adrenal Fatigue with a critical and balanced perspective. If you suspect you have Adrenal Fatigue or are experiencing any of the symptoms mentioned above, it is crucial to consult a healthcare professional for a comprehensive evaluation and appropriate diagnosis. A thorough assessment can help rule out other medical conditions and ensure the most appropriate treatment plan is implemented to address your specific health needs.

1.2 Causes and Risk Factors of Adrenal Fatigue Syndrome

The concept of Adrenal Fatigue Syndrome suggests that chronic stress and its effects on the adrenal glands and the HPA axis are the primary drivers of this condition. While the validity of Adrenal Fatigue remains a subject of debate in the medical community, some factors are believed to contribute to the development of symptoms associated with this condition. It's important to note that these factors might also be associated with other health issues, making it challenging to attribute symptoms solely to Adrenal Fatigue.

Potential Causes of Adrenal Fatigue:

1. Chronic Stress: Prolonged exposure to physical, emotional, or psychological stress can place an increased demand on the adrenal glands to produce stress hormones like cortisol and adrenaline. Over time, this constant demand may lead to dysregulation of the HPA

axis and impact the body's ability to manage stress effectively.

2. Lifestyle Factors: Poor sleep habits, unhealthy dietary choices, lack of exercise, and a sedentary lifestyle can contribute to overall stress on the body, potentially affecting adrenal function.

3. Emotional and Mental Stress: Emotional trauma, anxiety, and unresolved psychological issues may trigger chronic stress responses, influencing adrenal gland activity.

4. Dietary Habits: Consuming excessive amounts of caffeine, sugar, and processed foods might strain the adrenal glands and exacerbate symptoms.

5. Infections and Illness: Chronic infections or long-term illness can

place additional stress on the body and contribute to adrenal imbalances.

6. Medical Treatments: Certain medical treatments, such as long-term corticosteroid use, can affect adrenal function and lead to symptoms similar to Adrenal Fatigue.

7. Environmental Toxins: Exposure to environmental toxins and pollutants may impact overall health and potentially contribute to adrenal dysregulation.

Risk Factors:

While anyone can experience stress-related symptoms, some factors may increase the likelihood of developing Adrenal Fatigue Syndrome:

1. High-Stress Lifestyle: Individuals who experience chronic stress due to work, family, or personal reasons may be at higher risk.

2. History of Trauma: Past traumatic experiences or ongoing emotional stress may contribute to HPA axis dysregulation.

3. Poor Sleep Patterns: Sleep deprivation or irregular sleep patterns can disrupt the body's natural stress response and cortisol production.

4. Unhealthy Diet: A diet high in processed foods, sugar, and caffeine might impact adrenal health.

5. Lack of Social Support: Limited social support or weak coping mechanisms can contribute to chronic stress.

6. Medical Conditions: Certain medical conditions, such as autoimmune disorders, chronic infections, or allergies, may increase the risk of experiencing symptoms similar to Adrenal Fatigue.

1.3 Recognizing the Symptoms of Adrenal Fatigue Syndrome

The symptoms associated with Adrenal Fatigue can vary from person to person, and not everyone will experience the same set of symptoms. Additionally, many of these symptoms can be seen in other health conditions, which makes diagnosing Adrenal Fatigue challenging. However, some common signs and symptoms attributed to Adrenal Fatigue include:

1. Chronic Fatigue: Persistent, unexplained fatigue and a feeling of being "burned out" even after sufficient rest.

2. Sleep Disturbances: Difficulty falling asleep, staying asleep, or waking up feeling unrefreshed.

3. Stress and Anxiety: Heightened sensitivity to stress and difficulty coping with daily challenges.

4. Brain Fog and Memory Issues: Difficulty concentrating, memory lapses, and reduced mental clarity.

5. Low Energy and Motivation: Decreased energy levels and lack of enthusiasm for activities.

6. Digestive Problems: Bloating, indigestion, or other gastrointestinal discomfort.

7. Changes in Weight: Unexplained weight gain or difficulty losing weight.

8. Low Blood Pressure: A drop in blood pressure, leading to dizziness or lightheadedness.

9. Sensitivity to Cold: Feeling excessively cold, especially in the extremities.

10. Reduced Immune Function: Frequent illnesses and prolonged recovery periods.

Recognizing these symptoms can be a starting point for identifying potential issues, but it's crucial to consult with a qualified healthcare professional for an accurate diagnosis and appropriate management. Due to the overlap with other health conditions, comprehensive evaluation and ruling out other possible causes are essential for determining the most suitable treatment approach.

CHAPTER 2

Understanding the Adrenal Glands and their Functions

2.1 Anatomy of the Adrenal Glands

The adrenal glands are small, triangular-shaped endocrine glands located on top of each kidney. Despite their small size, these glands play a vital role in regulating various physiological processes throughout the body. Each adrenal gland is composed of two main parts: the adrenal cortex and the adrenal medulla.

- Adrenal Cortex: The outer layer of the adrenal gland is known as the adrenal cortex. It synthesizes and releases essential steroid hormones, including glucocorticoids (such as cortisol), mineralocorticoids (such as aldosterone), and small amounts of sex hormones (e.g., testosterone and estrogen). These hormones are critical for maintaining proper blood pressure, electrolyte balance, metabolism, and immune response.

- Adrenal Medulla: The inner part of the adrenal gland is called the adrenal medulla. It is responsible for producing and releasing catecholamines, which include adrenaline (epinephrine) and noradrenaline (norepinephrine). These hormones are involved in the body's stress response and play a crucial role in the "fight or flight" reaction when faced with a perceived threat or stressor.

The regulation of adrenal hormones is intricately controlled by a complex feedback system involving the hypothalamus and the pituitary gland, known as the hypothalamic-pituitary-adrenal (HPA) axis. When the body experiences stress or requires an increased hormone release, the HPA axis is activated to ensure an appropriate response.

2.2 The Role of Adrenal Hormones

Adrenal hormones play diverse and essential roles in the body, influencing various physiological processes and helping the body maintain balance, or homeostasis. Here are some of the key functions of the major adrenal hormones:

- Cortisol: Often referred to as the "stress hormone," cortisol helps the body respond to stress by increasing blood sugar levels, suppressing the immune system, and promoting the breakdown of fats, carbohydrates, and proteins for energy. Cortisol also has anti-inflammatory effects and assists in regulating blood pressure.

- Aldosterone: This mineralocorticoid hormone is responsible for maintaining the body's fluid balance and electrolyte levels, particularly by increasing the reabsorption of sodium and water in the kidneys while promoting the excretion of potassium.

- Adrenaline (Epinephrine) and Noradrenaline (Norepinephrine): These catecholamines are involved in the "fight or flight" response to stress. They increase heart rate, boost energy production, and redirect blood flow to essential organs, preparing the body to respond to perceived threats.

- Sex Hormones: While the adrenal glands produce smaller amounts of sex hormones compared to the gonads (testes in males and ovaries in females), they still play a role in supporting reproductive function and overall hormonal balance.

The secretion of these hormones is tightly regulated to ensure their appropriate levels within the body. When the adrenal glands function optimally, they contribute to overall health and well-being.

2.3 How Stress Affects Adrenal Function

When the body experiences stress, whether it's physical, emotional, or psychological, the HPA axis is activated to initiate the stress response. Here's a simplified overview of how stress affects adrenal function:

1. Perception of Stress: The brain's hypothalamus detects stressors and sends signals to the pituitary gland.

2. Pituitary Gland Response: The pituitary gland, in response to the hypothalamic signals, releases adrenocorticotropic hormone (ACTH) into the bloodstream.

3. ACTH Stimulates the Adrenal Cortex: ACTH travels through the bloodstream and stimulates the

adrenal cortex to produce and release cortisol and other glucocorticoids.

4. Cortisol Release: Cortisol levels rise in the blood, helping the body cope with stress by increasing blood sugar levels, suppressing non-essential bodily functions (like digestion and reproductive processes), and promoting energy availability for the muscles and brain.

5. Fight or Flight Response: In parallel, the adrenal medulla releases adrenaline and noradrenaline, which rapidly increase heart rate, boost energy, and redirect blood flow to support immediate physical action.

Once the stressor diminishes, the HPA axis feedback system works to reduce cortisol and catecholamine production, returning the body to its normal state of balance.

While this stress response is a natural and adaptive mechanism, chronic or prolonged stress can lead to persistent activation of the HPA axis, causing imbalances in adrenal hormones. Over time, this dysregulation may be associated with symptoms commonly attributed to Adrenal Fatigue Syndrome. It is essential to recognize that chronic stress can have widespread effects on overall health and well-being, and managing stress effectively is crucial for maintaining adrenal health.

CHAPTER 3

Diagnosing Adrenal Fatigue Syndrome

3.1 Medical History and Physical Examination

Diagnosing Adrenal Fatigue Syndrome can be challenging, as the term itself is controversial, and the symptoms associated with it overlap with many other health conditions. However, a thorough medical history and physical examination are essential initial steps in the diagnostic process.

During the medical history, the healthcare provider will ask detailed questions about the patient's symptoms, their duration, and any potential triggers or stressors. They will inquire about the patient's lifestyle, sleep patterns, dietary habits, and stress levels. Additionally, the healthcare provider will review the patient's medical history, family history, and any past or ongoing medical conditions.

The physical examination may include a general assessment of the patient's overall health, vital signs (such as blood pressure and heart rate), and a focused examination of specific body systems related to the reported symptoms. The goal of the physical examination is to identify any potential physical signs that may suggest adrenal dysfunction.

3.2 Saliva and Blood Tests for Adrenal Hormones:

Measuring adrenal hormones is a common approach used by some practitioners to evaluate adrenal function and potentially support the diagnosis of Adrenal Fatigue Syndrome. Two primary methods for assessing adrenal hormones are saliva testing and blood testing.

- Saliva Testing: Saliva tests are non-invasive and may be used to measure cortisol levels at multiple time points throughout the day. This approach is based on the understanding that cortisol levels follow a diurnal (daily) pattern, with higher levels in the morning and lower levels in the evening. Saliva testing may provide insights into cortisol fluctuations, which can be useful in assessing HPA axis function.

- Blood Testing: Blood tests can also measure cortisol levels, as well as other hormones produced by the adrenal glands, such as aldosterone and DHEA (dehydroepiandrosterone). Blood tests are typically taken at specific times, as cortisol levels can fluctuate throughout the day. Blood tests offer a more comprehensive assessment of adrenal hormone levels compared to saliva tests.

It is important to note that there is controversy within the medical community regarding the accuracy and clinical relevance of saliva testing for assessing adrenal function. Some healthcare professionals question its reliability, while others find value in its use as part of a broader evaluation.

3.3 Differentiating Adrenal Fatigue from Other Conditions

Since the symptoms associated with Adrenal Fatigue overlap with those of many other health conditions, it is crucial to differentiate Adrenal Fatigue from other potential causes. Conditions with similar symptoms may include chronic fatigue syndrome, depression, thyroid disorders, anemia, sleep disorders, and various hormonal imbalances, among others.

To differentiate Adrenal Fatigue from other conditions, the healthcare provider may:

- Rule Out Other Medical Conditions: The healthcare provider will perform specific tests or screenings to rule out other potential medical causes of the patient's symptoms. This may involve blood tests, imaging studies, or referrals to specialists.

- Comprehensive Evaluation: A comprehensive evaluation of the patient's medical history, symptoms, physical examination, and test results helps the healthcare provider form a holistic understanding of the patient's health status.

- Consideration of Stressors: The healthcare provider will assess the patient's exposure to stress and evaluate how stress may be contributing to the reported symptoms.

- Collaboration with Specialists: In some cases, collaboration with other healthcare specialists, such as endocrinologists or psychiatrists, may be necessary for a comprehensive evaluation.

It is essential for patients and healthcare providers to approach the diagnosis of Adrenal Fatigue with caution and an open mind. In cases where symptoms are persistent and unclear, it may be helpful to consider multiple factors that could be contributing to the patient's health concerns. The focus should be on addressing the patient's overall well-being, regardless of whether a specific diagnosis of Adrenal Fatigue is made.

CHAPTER 4

Lifestyle Changes for Managing Adrenal Fatigue

4.1 Stress Management Techniques

Since stress is believed to be a significant factor in Adrenal Fatigue Syndrome, effective stress management techniques are essential for managing this condition. Here are some strategies to help reduce and cope with stress:

- Mindfulness and Meditation: Practices such as mindfulness meditation, deep breathing exercises, and progressive muscle relaxation can help promote relaxation and reduce the body's stress response.

- Yoga and Tai Chi: These mind-body practices combine physical movement with breath control and meditation, fostering a sense of calm and promoting overall well-being.

- Time Management: Learning to prioritize tasks, set realistic goals, and avoid overcommitting can help reduce stress and prevent feeling overwhelmed.

- Establishing Boundaries: Setting boundaries in personal and professional relationships can prevent unnecessary stress and support a healthier balance in life.

- Social Support: Engaging with friends, family, or support groups can provide emotional support and help individuals cope with stress more effectively.

- Hobbies and Leisure Activities: Engaging in activities that bring joy and relaxation can serve as a valuable stress-relief outlet.

4.2 Sleep Optimization

Restorative sleep is crucial for overall health and adrenal function. Adopting healthy sleep habits can help improve sleep quality and support adrenal recovery:

- Maintain a Consistent Sleep Schedule: Try to go to bed and wake up at the same time each day, even on weekends.

- Create a Relaxing Bedtime
  Routine: Establish a calming
  routine before bedtime, such as
  reading, taking a warm bath, or
  practicing relaxation techniques.

- Limit Stimulants: Avoid caffeine
  and other stimulants close to
  bedtime, as they can interfere with
  falling asleep.

- Create a Sleep-Friendly
  Environment: Ensure the bedroom
  is quiet, dark, and at a comfortable
  temperature to promote better
  sleep.

- Limit Screen Time: Avoid
  electronic devices, such as
  smartphones and computers, at
  least an hour before bedtime, as
  the blue light can disrupt the sleep-
  wake cycle.

- Manage Stress: Stress reduction techniques (mentioned in section 4.1) can also help improve sleep quality.

4.3 Balanced Nutrition and Dietary Recommendations

A balanced and nutrient-rich diet is essential for supporting adrenal health and overall well-being:

- Balanced Meals: Aim to include a variety of whole foods, including fruits, vegetables, whole grains, lean proteins, and healthy fats in your diet.

- Avoid Skipping Meals: Skipping meals can lead to drops in blood sugar levels, which may trigger stress responses.

- Limit Sugary and Processed Foods: High-sugar and processed foods can lead to energy spikes and crashes, impacting overall energy levels and mood.

- Monitor Caffeine Intake: Limit caffeine consumption, as excessive amounts can contribute to increased stress and disrupt sleep.

- Stay Hydrated: Proper hydration is vital for maintaining bodily functions and supporting adrenal health.

4.4 Importance of Regular Exercise

Regular physical activity can have a positive impact on adrenal health and stress management:

- Choose Activities You Enjoy: Engage in exercises or physical activities that you find enjoyable, as this will increase your likelihood of sticking with the routine.

- Moderate Exercise: Aim for regular moderate-intensity activities, such as brisk walking, swimming, or cycling.

- Avoid Overexertion: Excessive or intense exercise can increase stress on the body and potentially worsen adrenal imbalances.

- Balance Rest and Activity: Ensure that you balance exercise with adequate rest and recovery.

- Mindful Movement: Mind-body practices like yoga and tai chi (mentioned in section 4.1) can be beneficial for both physical activity and stress reduction.

It's important to note that lifestyle changes alone may not be sufficient to address complex health issues. If you suspect you have Adrenal Fatigue or are experiencing persistent symptoms, consult a qualified healthcare professional for a comprehensive evaluation and personalized treatment plan. They can help determine the most appropriate approach to support your adrenal health and overall well-being.

CHAPTER 5

Herbal and Nutritional Supplements for Adrenal Support

5.1 Adaptogenic Herbs

Adaptogenic herbs are a class of botanicals known for their ability to help the body adapt to stress and promote balance within various physiological systems. They are believed to support adrenal function and may be helpful for individuals experiencing Adrenal Fatigue symptoms. Some commonly used adaptogenic herbs include:

- Ashwagandha (Withania somnifera): Ashwagandha is one of the most well-known adaptogens. It may help reduce stress and anxiety, support the adrenal glands, and improve overall energy levels.

- Rhodiola (Rhodiola rosea): Rhodiola is believed to enhance stress resilience, improve mental and physical performance, and reduce fatigue.

- Holy Basil (Ocimum sanctum): Also known as Tulsi, Holy Basil is used traditionally to promote relaxation and support the body's response to stress.

- Ginseng (Panax ginseng): Ginseng is an adaptogenic herb that may help improve stamina, reduce fatigue, and support adrenal health.

- Licorice Root (Glycyrrhiza glabra): Licorice root is thought to have adrenal-supporting properties and may help maintain cortisol balance.

It's important to consult with a healthcare professional or qualified herbalist before using adaptogenic herbs, as they may interact with certain medications or have contraindications for certain health conditions. Additionally, individual responses to herbal supplements can vary, so it's crucial to use them under proper guidance.

5.2 Vitamins and Minerals for Adrenal Health

Certain vitamins and minerals play essential roles in supporting adrenal function and overall well-being. Some of these include:

- Vitamin C: Vitamin C is a potent antioxidant that supports the immune system and helps mitigate the effects of stress on the body.

- B Vitamins: B vitamins, particularly B5 (pantothenic acid) and B6 (pyridoxine), are involved in adrenal hormone production and energy metabolism.

- Magnesium: Magnesium is essential for muscle function, relaxation, and stress management.

- Zinc: Zinc plays a role in immune function and hormone regulation, supporting overall adrenal health.

- Vitamin D: Adequate vitamin D levels are important for immune function and mood regulation, which can indirectly impact adrenal health.

- Selenium: Selenium is involved in thyroid hormone conversion and supports the body's antioxidant defense system.

It's important to obtain these vitamins and minerals through a balanced diet whenever possible. However, in cases of deficiency or under guidance from a healthcare professional, supplementation may be considered.

5.3 Recommended Dosages and Precautions

The dosages and specific formulations of herbal and nutritional supplements for adrenal support may vary depending on individual needs, health status, and the presence of any medical conditions. It is crucial to work with a qualified healthcare professional, such as a naturopathic doctor, functional medicine practitioner, or registered dietitian, before starting any supplementation regimen.

Here are some general precautions to consider:

- Individual Variations: Each person's response to supplements can differ, and what works for one individual may not be suitable for another. Customized recommendations are essential.

- Interactions: Some supplements may interact with medications or other supplements, so it's important to disclose all medications and supplements you are taking to your healthcare provider.

- Quality and Safety: Choose reputable brands that adhere to good manufacturing practices (GMP) and third-party testing for quality and purity.

- Dosage: Follow the recommended dosages provided by your healthcare professional and avoid exceeding the recommended amounts unless specifically advised.

- Duration: Use supplements as part of a comprehensive approach to adrenal support, which may include lifestyle changes, stress management, and dietary adjustments.

Herbal and nutritional supplements are not meant to replace a balanced diet or any prescribed medications. They are intended to complement a comprehensive approach to supporting adrenal health and overall well-being. Always seek professional guidance to tailor a supplementation plan that suits your specific needs and health goals.

CHAPTER 6

Prescription Medications for Adrenal Fatigue

6.1 Corticosteroids and their Use

Corticosteroids are a class of prescription medications that mimic the effects of natural steroid hormones produced by the adrenal glands, such as cortisol. They have potent anti-inflammatory and immunosuppressive properties and are commonly prescribed to treat various medical conditions, including autoimmune disorders, allergic reactions, and inflammatory conditions.

In the context of Adrenal Fatigue, the use of corticosteroids is a subject of controversy. Adrenal Fatigue Syndrome implies that the adrenal glands are not functioning optimally and may have difficulty producing adequate cortisol levels. In severe cases of adrenal insufficiency, such as Addison's disease, cortisol replacement therapy with corticosteroids may be necessary to maintain essential bodily functions.

However, in cases where Adrenal Fatigue is considered a milder dysfunction, the use of corticosteroids is generally not recommended. Using these medications for mild adrenal imbalances may suppress the body's natural feedback mechanisms and further compromise adrenal function in the long run.

It's important to emphasize that the use of corticosteroids should only be considered under the guidance and prescription of a qualified healthcare professional, and only in cases of diagnosed adrenal insufficiency or specific medical conditions that warrant their use.

6.2 Risks and Benefits of Medication

The use of prescription medications, including corticosteroids, should always be carefully weighed for their potential risks and benefits. Some considerations include:

Benefits:

- Corticosteroids can be life-saving for individuals with severe adrenal insufficiency, such as Addison's disease, by providing essential hormones that the body cannot produce on its own.

- These medications are highly effective in treating acute inflammatory conditions, allergic reactions, and certain autoimmune diseases.

- In specific medical situations, corticosteroids may provide significant relief from symptoms and improve overall quality of life.

Risks:

- Long-term use of corticosteroids can lead to a range of side effects, including weight gain, bone loss (osteoporosis), increased blood pressure, elevated blood sugar levels, and increased risk of infections.

- Abruptly stopping or rapidly tapering corticosteroids after long-term use can lead to withdrawal symptoms and adrenal insufficiency, as the body's natural cortisol production may be suppressed.

- Corticosteroids can interact with other medications, and their use may be contraindicated in certain medical conditions.

- Prolonged use of corticosteroids can suppress the immune system, making individuals more susceptible to infections.

6.3 Monitoring and Adjusting Treatment

For individuals prescribed corticosteroids for adrenal

insufficiency or other medical conditions, close monitoring by a healthcare professional is essential. Regular follow-up appointments and blood tests may be necessary to assess hormone levels, monitor for side effects, and make adjustments to the treatment plan as needed.

Patients should never discontinue or adjust their corticosteroid dosage without consulting their healthcare provider, as abrupt changes can lead to serious health complications.

If you suspect you have Adrenal Fatigue or are experiencing symptoms, it's important to seek the guidance of a healthcare professional. They can provide a comprehensive evaluation, determine the most appropriate course of action, and discuss potential treatment options tailored to your specific needs and health condition. Remember that managing adrenal health often involves a holistic approach that includes lifestyle changes, stress management, dietary adjustments, and potential complementary therapies, and prescription medications should only be considered when medically necessary and prescribed by a qualified healthcare professional.

CHAPTER 7

Complementary Therapies for Adrenal Fatigue

7.1 Acupuncture and Acupressure

Acupuncture and acupressure are traditional Chinese medicine practices that involve stimulating specific points on the body to promote energy flow and balance. Both therapies are based on the concept of qi (pronounced "chee"), the vital energy that flows through meridians or channels in the body.

7.1.1 Acupuncture

During acupuncture, thin, sterile needles are inserted into specific acupuncture points along the meridians. The goal is to regulate the flow of qi, which is believed to influence various bodily functions and promote overall well-being. Acupuncture is often used to help reduce stress, improve energy levels, and support the body's natural healing processes.

7.1.2 Acupressure

Acupressure involves applying pressure to the same acupuncture points, but without the use of needles. Instead, finger pressure, massage, or specialized tools are used to stimulate these points. Acupressure can be a gentle and non-invasive alternative for those who may be uncomfortable with acupuncture needles.

While there is limited scientific research specifically on acupuncture and acupressure for Adrenal Fatigue, some studies suggest that these therapies may have a positive impact on stress reduction and overall well-being. They are generally considered safe when performed by qualified practitioners.

7.2 Massage Therapy

Massage therapy involves the manipulation of soft tissues, muscles, and connective tissues to promote relaxation, reduce muscle tension, and improve circulation. Several types of massage techniques can be beneficial for individuals with Adrenal Fatigue:

- Swedish Massage: This gentle and relaxing massage uses long, flowing strokes and kneading to

promote relaxation and stress
reduction.

- Deep Tissue Massage: Deep tissue
massage targets deeper layers of
muscle tissue to release tension
and knots. It may help relieve
muscle soreness and improve
flexibility.

- Aromatherapy Massage: This
massage combines massage
techniques with the use of essential
oils to enhance relaxation and
promote a sense of well-being.

- Reflexology: Reflexology is a type
of massage that focuses on specific
points on the feet, hands, or ears
that correspond to various organs
and systems in the body. It is
believed to help stimulate energy
flow and support overall health.

Massage therapy can be an effective complementary therapy for Adrenal Fatigue by promoting relaxation, reducing stress, and improving sleep quality. It can also help alleviate muscle tension, which may be beneficial for individuals experiencing physical discomfort related to stress.

As with any complementary therapy, it's essential to consult a qualified and experienced practitioner. Massage therapy is generally safe for most people, but certain medical conditions or individual health considerations may require specific modifications or precautions.

While complementary therapies can be valuable additions to an overall approach to managing Adrenal Fatigue, it's crucial to remember that they should not replace conventional medical care. A comprehensive treatment plan that includes lifestyle changes, stress management, proper nutrition, and, if needed, appropriate medical interventions, provides the best chance for supporting adrenal health and overall well-being. Always consult with a healthcare professional to determine the most suitable and safe approach for your specific health needs.

7.3 Yoga and Meditation

Yoga and meditation are mind-body practices that have been used for centuries to promote physical, mental, and emotional well-being. They are effective complementary therapies for managing stress and supporting adrenal health in individuals with Adrenal Fatigue.

7.3.1 Yoga

Yoga combines physical postures (asanas), breath control (pranayama), and meditation to create a holistic practice that helps reduce stress and promote relaxation. Regular practice of yoga can improve flexibility, balance, and strength while calming the mind and relieving tension. Certain yoga poses, such as gentle backbends and inversions, are believed to stimulate the adrenal glands and support adrenal health. Additionally, the focus on deep breathing during yoga helps activate the body's relaxation response, reducing the production of stress hormones.

7.3.2 Meditation

Meditation involves training the mind to focus on the present moment, promoting mindfulness and mental clarity. Various meditation techniques, such as mindfulness meditation, loving-kindness meditation, and transcendental meditation, can help reduce stress, anxiety, and negative thought patterns. By encouraging a sense of inner calm and emotional balance, meditation supports overall well-being and may help manage the effects of chronic stress on the body, including the adrenal glands.

Both yoga and meditation can be adapted to suit individual needs and abilities. They are generally considered safe for most people and can be practiced as part of a daily routine or during times of stress.

7.4 Biofeedback and Relaxation Techniques

Biofeedback is a therapeutic technique that helps individuals become more aware of their body's physiological responses, such as heart rate, blood pressure, and muscle tension. Through the use of specialized equipment, individuals can learn to control or change these responses to promote relaxation and stress reduction.

7.4.1 Relaxation Techniques

Various relaxation techniques, such as progressive muscle relaxation, guided imagery, and breathing exercises, can be incorporated into biofeedback sessions or used independently. These techniques help activate the body's relaxation response, which counteracts the stress response and supports adrenal health.

7.4.2 Biofeedback

Biofeedback sessions involve monitoring physiological responses, such as heart rate variability, skin temperature, or muscle tension, using electronic sensors. With the guidance of a biofeedback therapist, individuals learn to recognize stress-related physiological changes and are taught strategies to consciously influence these responses. The goal is to promote relaxation and self-regulation, which can be beneficial for managing stress-related conditions, including Adrenal Fatigue.

Biofeedback and relaxation techniques are generally safe and well-tolerated. They can empower individuals to take an active role in managing stress and promoting well-being.

It's important to remember that while complementary therapies can be beneficial, they should be used as part of a comprehensive approach to managing Adrenal Fatigue. This approach should include lifestyle changes, stress management, dietary adjustments, and, if needed, medical interventions. Always consult with a qualified healthcare professional to ensure that these complementary therapies are suitable for your specific health needs and to receive guidance on incorporating them effectively into your overall treatment plan.

CHAPTER 8

Lifestyle Tips for Long-Term Adrenal Health

8.1 Creating a Supportive Environment

Creating a supportive environment is essential for long-term adrenal health. This involves making intentional changes in your daily life to reduce stress and promote overall well-being. Here are some tips to create a supportive environment:

- Set Boundaries: Learn to say no to commitments that may overwhelm you and prioritize self-care.

- Surround Yourself with Support:
  Build a network of supportive
  friends, family, or a community
  that you can rely on during
  challenging times.

- Declutter: Organize your living
  space to create a calming and
  clutter-free environment.

- Create a Relaxation Space:
  Designate a peaceful space in your
  home where you can practice
  relaxation techniques, such as
  meditation or deep breathing.

- Limit Exposure to Stressors:
  Identify and minimize exposure to
  unnecessary stressors in your life,
  whether they are related to work,
  relationships, or other external
  factors.

8.2 Building Resilience to Stress

Building resilience to stress is crucial for long-term adrenal health. Resilience involves developing coping skills and strategies to adapt to stress in a healthy way. Here are some tips to build resilience:

- Practice Mindfulness: Stay present and focused on the current moment, rather than dwelling on past regrets or worrying about the future.

- Cultivate Positive Thinking: Challenge negative thought patterns and practice gratitude to shift your perspective.

- Engage in Stress-Relieving Activities: Engage in activities that bring you joy and relaxation, such as spending time in nature, pursuing hobbies, or spending time with loved ones.

- Prioritize Self-Care: Make time for self-care activities that nourish your mind, body, and spirit.

- Seek Professional Support: If you're struggling with chronic stress or finding it challenging to build resilience, consider seeking support from a therapist or counselor.

8.3 Monitoring Progress and Identifying Triggers

Monitoring your progress and identifying triggers that exacerbate your symptoms can help you make informed decisions about your lifestyle and treatment plan. Here are some tips for monitoring and identifying triggers:

- Keep a Journal: Keep a daily journal to record your symptoms, stress levels, dietary habits, and any notable events. This can help you identify patterns and potential triggers.

- Track Sleep Patterns: Monitor your sleep quality and patterns, as sleep is essential for adrenal health.

- Observe Stress Responses: Pay attention to your body's stress responses and note how different stressors affect you.

- Experiment with Lifestyle Changes: Make gradual lifestyle changes and observe how they impact your well-being over time.

- Work with a Healthcare Professional: Share your journal and observations with your healthcare provider to collaboratively assess progress and make necessary adjustments to your treatment plan.

Long-term adrenal health is a journey that requires patience and commitment to making sustainable lifestyle changes. It's important to work with a qualified healthcare professional who can provide personalized guidance and support throughout this process.

In addition to the lifestyle tips mentioned above, consider implementing the lifestyle changes, stress management techniques, dietary recommendations, and complementary therapies discussed in earlier sections to support your overall

adrenal health. With a comprehensive
and individualized approach, you can
foster long-term well-being and
resilience to stress.

CHAPTER 9

Adrenal Fatigue in Special Populations

9.1 Adrenal Fatigue in Women

Adrenal Fatigue is a condition that can affect people of all genders, but there are specific considerations for women due to their unique hormonal fluctuations and life stages. Several factors may contribute to Adrenal Fatigue in women:

1. Hormonal Changes: Women experience hormonal fluctuations throughout their menstrual cycles, during pregnancy, and in perimenopause and menopause.

These fluctuations can impact adrenal function and contribute to increased stress on the body.

2. Pregnancy: Pregnancy places additional demands on a woman's body, including increased cortisol production to support fetal development. This can put strain on the adrenal glands, especially if the woman is already experiencing stress or other health challenges.

3. Postpartum Period: After childbirth, women may experience sleep disruptions, increased stress, and hormonal changes, which can affect adrenal health during the postpartum period.

4. Perimenopause and Menopause: As women approach menopause, hormonal imbalances can become more pronounced, potentially

impacting adrenal function. Changes in estrogen and progesterone levels can contribute to increased stress responses.

5. Polycystic Ovary Syndrome (PCOS): Women with PCOS may have imbalances in sex hormones and insulin, which can affect adrenal function and lead to symptoms resembling Adrenal Fatigue.

6. Thyroid Conditions: Women are more susceptible to thyroid disorders, and thyroid function is closely connected to adrenal health. Adrenal imbalances can influence thyroid function, and vice versa.

7. Stressful Life Events: Women may face specific stressors related to family, career, or societal

expectations, which can contribute to Adrenal Fatigue.

Managing Adrenal Fatigue in women requires a tailored approach that considers their unique hormonal fluctuations and life stages. Lifestyle changes, stress management techniques, and appropriate dietary adjustments can play a crucial role in supporting adrenal health. Women experiencing significant symptoms or concerns related to adrenal function should seek guidance from healthcare professionals who specialize in hormonal health and integrative medicine.

As with any health condition, it's essential to prioritize self-care and seek professional support when needed to maintain overall well-being. Women should also remember to advocate for their health and communicate openly with their healthcare providers about any symptoms or concerns they may have.

9.2 Adrenal Fatigue in Men

Adrenal Fatigue can also affect men, although it is often discussed more in the context of women's health. Men, like women, can experience imbalances in adrenal function and the associated symptoms related to stress and fatigue. Some considerations for Adrenal Fatigue in men include:

1. Lifestyle and Stress: Men may experience stress due to various factors, including work, family responsibilities, financial pressures, and societal

expectations. Chronic stress can have a significant impact on adrenal health.

2. Hormonal Changes: While women experience more pronounced hormonal fluctuations due to menstrual cycles, men also have hormonal changes as they age. Declining testosterone levels, which can occur with age (andropause), can affect adrenal function and the body's stress response.

3. Sleep Disruptions: Poor sleep habits, sleep disorders, or irregular sleep schedules can negatively affect adrenal health in men, just as in women.

4. Work-Life Balance: Balancing career demands, personal life, and

self-care can influence stress levels in men and impact adrenal health.

5. Diet and Nutrition: Poor dietary choices and inadequate nutrition can contribute to stress on the body and may affect adrenal function in men.

6. Exercise and Physical Activity: Overtraining or excessive physical activity without adequate recovery can lead to increased stress and potentially impact adrenal health in men.

7. Health Conditions: Certain health conditions, such as obesity, diabetes, and cardiovascular diseases, can influence adrenal function and exacerbate Adrenal Fatigue symptoms in men.

Managing Adrenal Fatigue in men requires a comprehensive approach that addresses lifestyle factors, stress management, and overall well-being. Regular exercise, balanced nutrition, quality sleep, and stress reduction techniques are key components of supporting adrenal health in men.

Men experiencing symptoms related to Adrenal Fatigue should seek guidance from healthcare professionals who can help identify potential underlying causes and provide appropriate support. Just like with women, it's essential for men to prioritize their health and well-being, and communicate openly with their healthcare providers about any concerns they may have. Adrenal Fatigue is a condition that can be effectively managed with lifestyle adjustments and proper care.

CHAPTER 10

Seeking Professional Help and Finding the Right Specialist

10.1 Choosing the Right Healthcare Provider

When dealing with potential health concerns like Adrenal Fatigue, finding the right healthcare provider is crucial for accurate diagnosis and effective treatment. Here are some steps to help you choose the right healthcare provider:

1. Primary Care Physician: Start by scheduling an appointment with your primary care physician

(PCP). They can assess your symptoms, perform initial tests, and refer you to specialists if necessary. PCPs are trained to manage a wide range of health conditions and can be a valuable resource in the diagnostic process.

2. Seek Recommendations: Ask friends, family members, or colleagues for recommendations of healthcare providers they trust. Personal referrals can provide valuable insights into the quality of care provided by a specific doctor.

3. Research Credentials: Look for healthcare providers with relevant credentials, board certifications, and affiliations with reputable medical organizations. Check their educational background and specialties to ensure they have

expertise in dealing with adrenal and endocrine-related issues.

4. Consider Specializations: Adrenal health is often related to endocrine health. Consider seeking care from an endocrinologist, who specializes in diagnosing and treating conditions related to hormones and glands, including the adrenal glands. Integrative or functional medicine practitioners may also have expertise in managing Adrenal Fatigue through a holistic approach.

5. Experience: Look for healthcare providers with experience in diagnosing and treating adrenal disorders or related conditions. Experienced practitioners may have encountered a broader range of cases and can offer more nuanced insights.

6. Patient Reviews: Read patient reviews and testimonials online to gather information about the experiences of others with a particular healthcare provider. While individual experiences may vary, positive feedback can be a good sign.

7. Communication Style: Consider your communication preferences. Choose a healthcare provider who listens to your concerns, takes time to explain treatment options, and involves you in the decision-making process.

8. Insurance Coverage: Check if the healthcare provider accepts your health insurance plan to minimize out-of-pocket expenses.

9. Location and Accessibility: Consider the location of the

healthcare provider's office and their availability for appointments. Easy accessibility can make it more convenient for follow-up visits and ongoing care.

10. Trust Your Instincts: Trust your instincts and choose a healthcare provider with whom you feel comfortable and confident.

Managing Adrenal Fatigue may involve a combination of lifestyle changes, stress management, dietary adjustments, complementary therapies, and, if necessary, medical interventions. A multidisciplinary approach that involves both traditional and alternative medicine can be beneficial in supporting adrenal health and overall well-being.

Always be open and honest with your healthcare provider about your symptoms, concerns, and any complementary therapies you are exploring. This will help them provide you with the most comprehensive and personalized care plan possible. Adrenal health is a journey, and finding the right healthcare partner can make a significant difference in achieving optimal well-being.

10.2 Questions to Ask During Consultations

When consulting with a healthcare provider regarding potential Adrenal Fatigue or adrenal health concerns, asking the right questions can help you gain a better understanding of your condition and the proposed treatment plan. Here are some

questions to consider asking during
your consultations:

1. What are the possible causes of my
   symptoms, and could Adrenal
   Fatigue be a contributing factor?

2. What tests or assessments will you
   use to diagnose or rule out Adrenal
   Fatigue or other adrenal-related
   conditions?

3. Can you explain the treatment
   options available for addressing
   Adrenal Fatigue, and what are the
   potential benefits and risks of
   each?

4. Are there any lifestyle changes,
   stress management techniques, or
   dietary recommendations that can
   support my adrenal health?

5. How can I improve my sleep
   quality and address any sleep

disturbances related to adrenal health?

6. Are there any specific supplements, vitamins, or herbal remedies that could be beneficial for supporting my adrenal function?

7. If necessary, would you consider prescribing medications, such as corticosteroids, to manage my adrenal health? What are the potential side effects and long-term implications of such medications?

8. What other medical conditions might have similar symptoms to Adrenal Fatigue, and how will you differentiate and rule them out?

9. How often should I follow up with you for monitoring and adjustments to my treatment plan?

10. Can you recommend any complementary therapies, such as yoga, meditation, or biofeedback, to support my overall well-being and adrenal health?

11. What lifestyle modifications can I make to manage stress and promote adrenal health in the long term?

12. Are there any specific activities or behaviors that I should avoid to prevent exacerbating my symptoms?

13. Can you provide guidance on managing stress and avoiding burnout, especially in relation to my career and daily responsibilities?

14. How will you work with me to create a personalized treatment

plan that suits my individual needs
and health goals?

15. Are there any specific symptoms
that may indicate a need for
immediate medical attention or
evaluation?

Take notes during the consultation
and ask for any additional resources
or educational materials that can help
you better understand your condition.
A good healthcare provider will take
the time to address your questions and
concerns, and they will collaborate
with you to develop a comprehensive
and personalized plan for managing
Adrenal Fatigue and supporting your
overall well-being.

CHAPTER 11

How Long Does Recovery from Adrenal Fatigue Take?

The duration of recovery from Adrenal Fatigue can vary significantly from person to person, and there is no one-size-fits-all answer to this question. Adrenal Fatigue is a complex condition, and recovery depends on various factors, including the severity of the adrenal imbalances, the individual's overall health, lifestyle factors, and the effectiveness of the treatment plan.

Recovering from Adrenal Fatigue typically requires a comprehensive approach that includes lifestyle changes, stress management, dietary adjustments, and, in some cases, complementary therapies or medical interventions. Here are some factors that can influence the duration of recovery:

1. Severity of Adrenal Imbalance: The extent of adrenal dysfunction can impact the recovery timeline. Mild cases may respond more quickly to lifestyle changes, while severe cases or advanced stages of adrenal dysfunction may require more time to restore optimal adrenal function.

2. Individual Response: Each person's body responds differently to treatment. Some individuals may experience significant improvement within a few weeks, while others may require several months to notice substantial changes.

3. Adherence to Treatment Plan: Consistency and adherence to the recommended treatment plan are crucial for successful recovery. Making sustained lifestyle changes and following healthcare provider's guidance is essential for achieving positive outcomes.

4. Overall, Health: The presence of other underlying health conditions can influence the speed of recovery. Addressing any co-existing health issues is important

for supporting adrenal health and overall well-being.

5. Stress Management: Effectively managing stress is a key component of Adrenal Fatigue recovery. Individuals who proactively adopt stress-reducing practices often experience faster improvements.

6. Sleep Quality: Quality and restorative sleep are vital for adrenal recovery. Improving sleep habits can accelerate the healing process.

7. Complementary Therapies: Some individuals may benefit from incorporating complementary therapies, such as yoga, meditation, or acupuncture, to enhance recovery. These therapies

can contribute to overall well-
being and support adrenal health.

It's essential to have realistic expectations during the recovery process. Adrenal Fatigue is not a quick fix, and it may take several months or even longer for some individuals to achieve significant improvement. Patience, consistency, and open communication with healthcare providers are essential throughout the recovery journey.

As the body heals and adrenal function improves, individuals often experience a gradual reduction in symptoms and an increase in energy levels and overall well-being. It's important to work closely with qualified healthcare professionals who can guide you through the recovery process, monitor progress, and make necessary adjustments to your

treatment plan as needed. Remember
that everyone's healing journey is
unique, and focusing on long-term
health and wellness is key to
sustaining adrenal health over time.

CHAPTER 12

Empowering Yourself for Recovery

Empowering yourself for recovery
from Adrenal Fatigue is crucial to
achieve positive outcomes and
improve overall well-being. Taking an
active role in your healing journey
can make a significant difference in
the success of your recovery. Here are

some empowering steps to support your journey to adrenal health:

1. Educate Yourself: Learn about Adrenal Fatigue, its symptoms, causes, and potential treatment options. Understanding the condition empowers you to make informed decisions about your health and collaborate effectively with healthcare providers.

2. Seek Professional Guidance: Consult with qualified healthcare professionals who specialize in adrenal health, endocrinology, or functional medicine. A knowledgeable and experienced healthcare team can provide personalized guidance and support tailored to your needs.

3. Advocate for Your Health: Be proactive in seeking answers to

your questions and concerns during medical appointments. Speak up about your symptoms, treatment preferences, and any challenges you face during your recovery.

4. Embrace Lifestyle Changes: Make positive lifestyle changes to support adrenal health, including stress reduction, regular exercise, balanced nutrition, and adequate sleep. Consistency in these lifestyle modifications is essential for long-term well-being.

5. Manage Stress: Adopt stress management techniques that work for you, such as meditation, yoga, deep breathing exercises, or spending time in nature. Managing stress effectively can significantly impact your adrenal recovery.

6. Prioritize Self-Care: Make self-care a priority in your daily life. Set aside time for activities that bring you joy, relaxation, and emotional well-being.

7. Monitor Progress: Keep a journal to track your symptoms, progress, and any patterns you observe. This can help you and your healthcare provider assess the effectiveness of your treatment plan.

8. Build a Support Network: Surround yourself with supportive friends, family, or support groups who understand and encourage your healing journey.

9. Be Patient and Kind to Yourself: Recovery from Adrenal Fatigue is a process that takes time and effort. Be patient with yourself and avoid self-criticism. Celebrate

even small improvements along the way.

10. Embrace Complementary Therapies: Consider incorporating complementary therapies, such as acupuncture, massage, or biofeedback, to enhance your recovery journey. These therapies can complement conventional treatments and support overall well-being.

11. Set Realistic Goals: Set achievable and realistic goals for your recovery. Celebrate each milestone and focus on the progress you are making.

12. Trust Your Instincts: Listen to your body and trust your instincts. If something doesn't feel right or if you have concerns about your treatment plan, communicate

openly with your healthcare provider.

Every individual's healing journey is unique, and recovery from Adrenal Fatigue may take time. Embrace the process, stay committed to your well-being, and seek the support you need to empower yourself throughout the recovery process. With dedication and self-compassion, you can take charge of your health and work towards restoring adrenal balance and overall vitality.